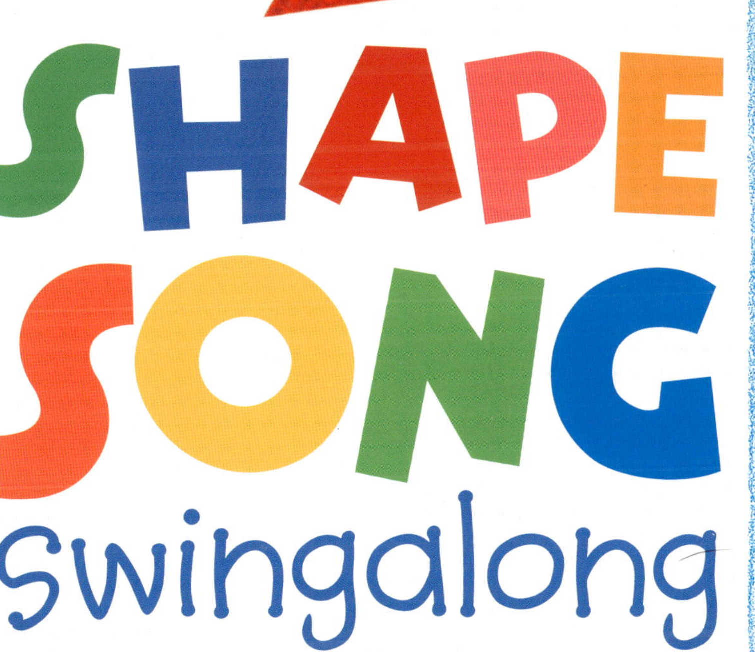

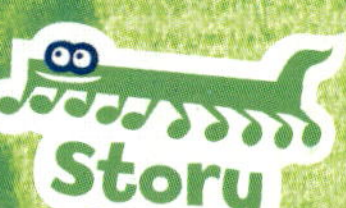

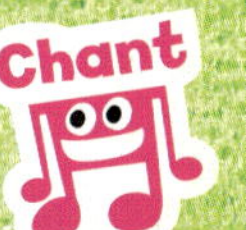

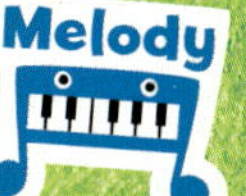

Written and sung by
STEVESONGS

Illustrated by
DAVID SIM

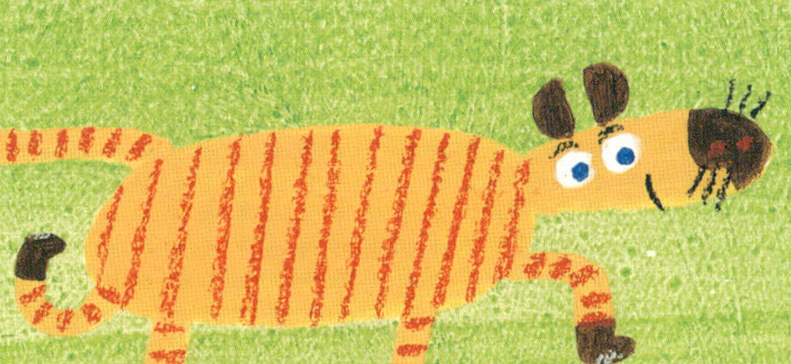

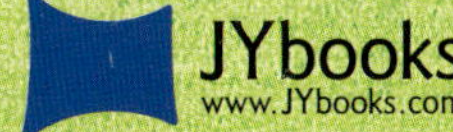

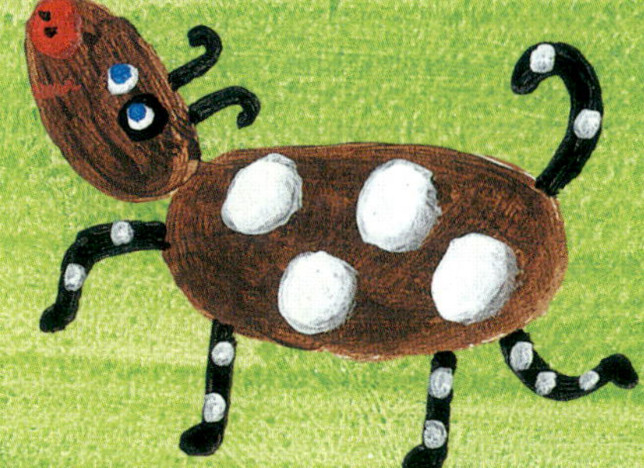

I have a shape collection and I use it to create
Anything I want to see or be or do or make.
Is it work? Is it play? Is it music? Is it art?

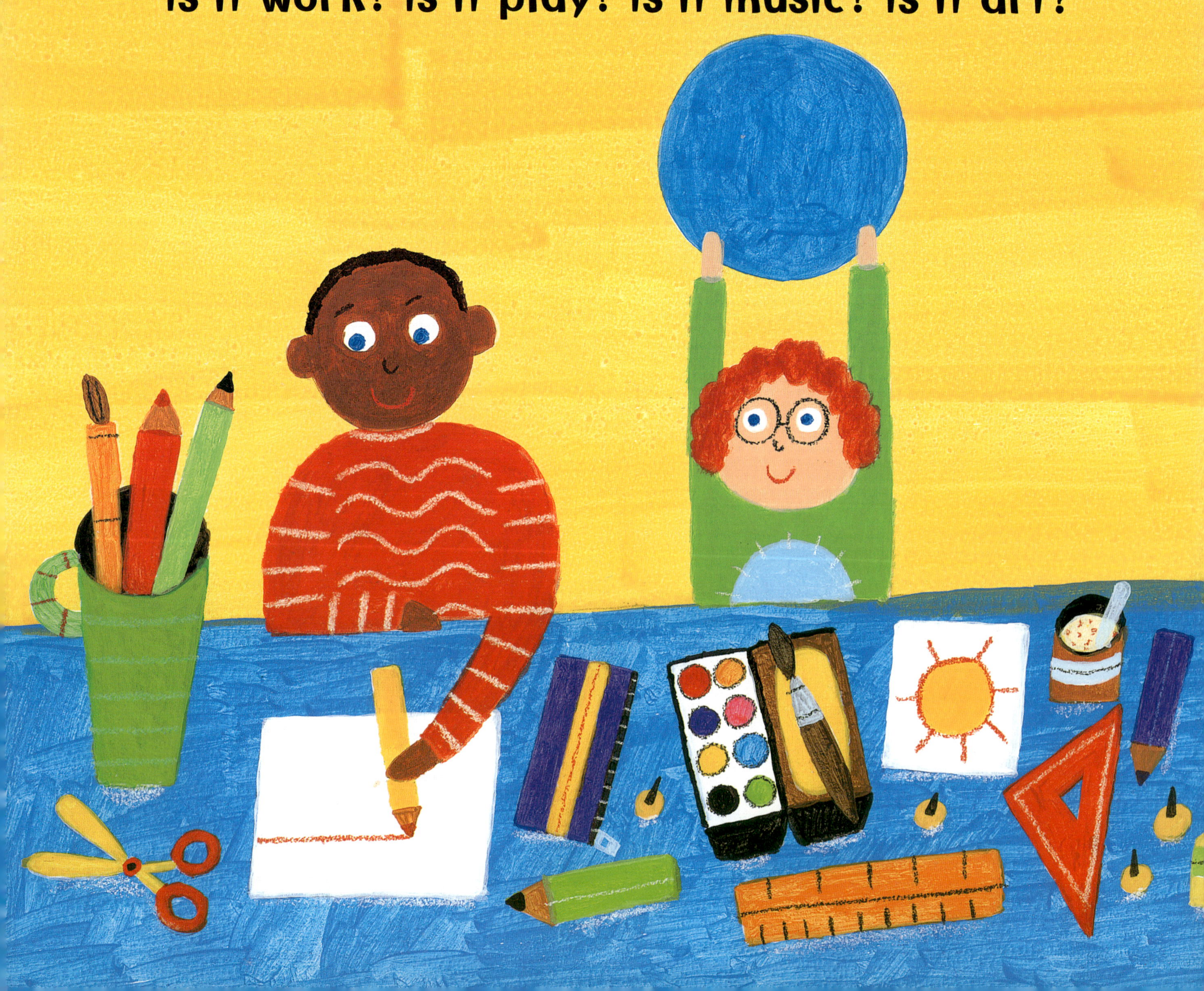

With my shape collection all I need to do is start

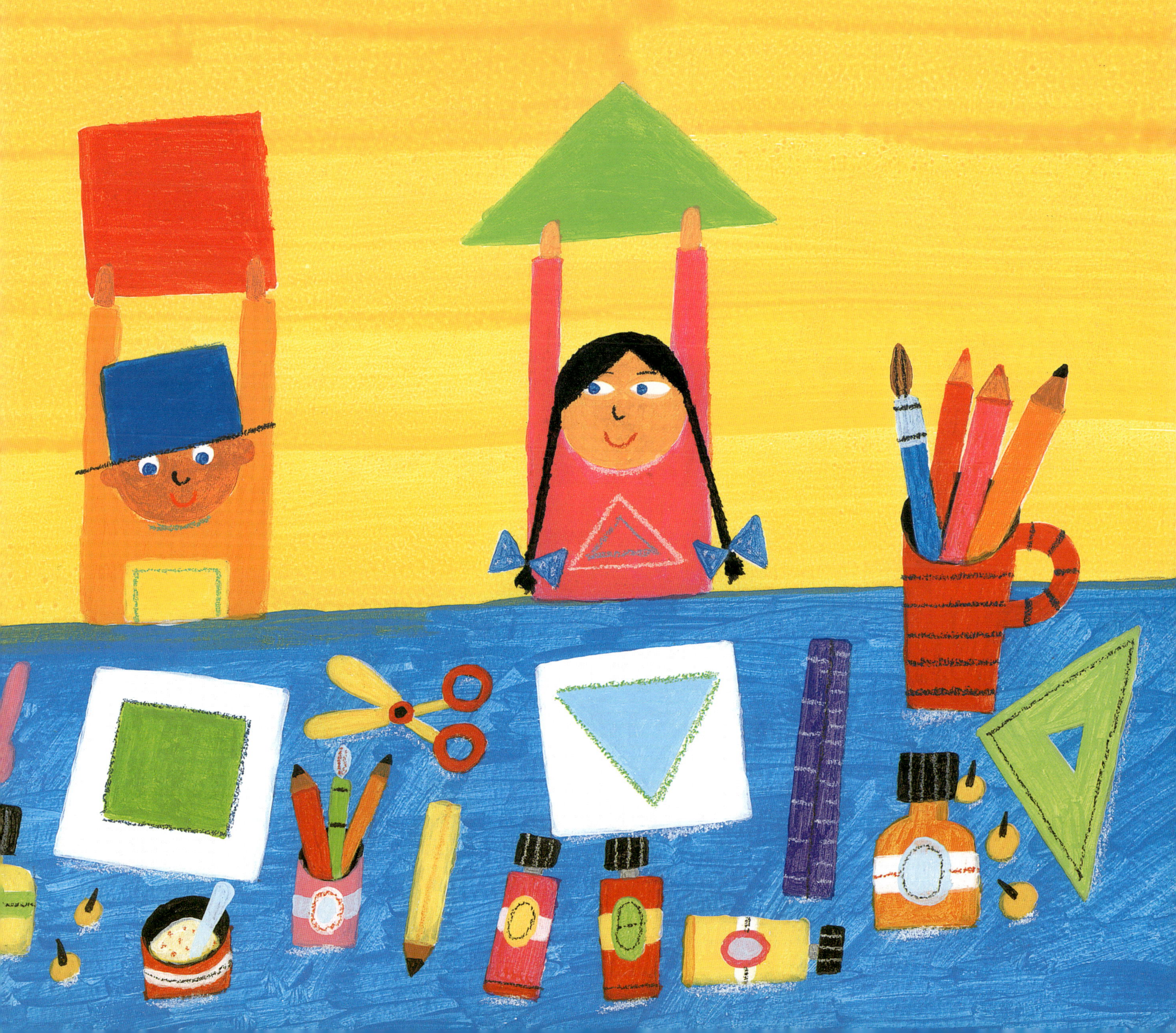

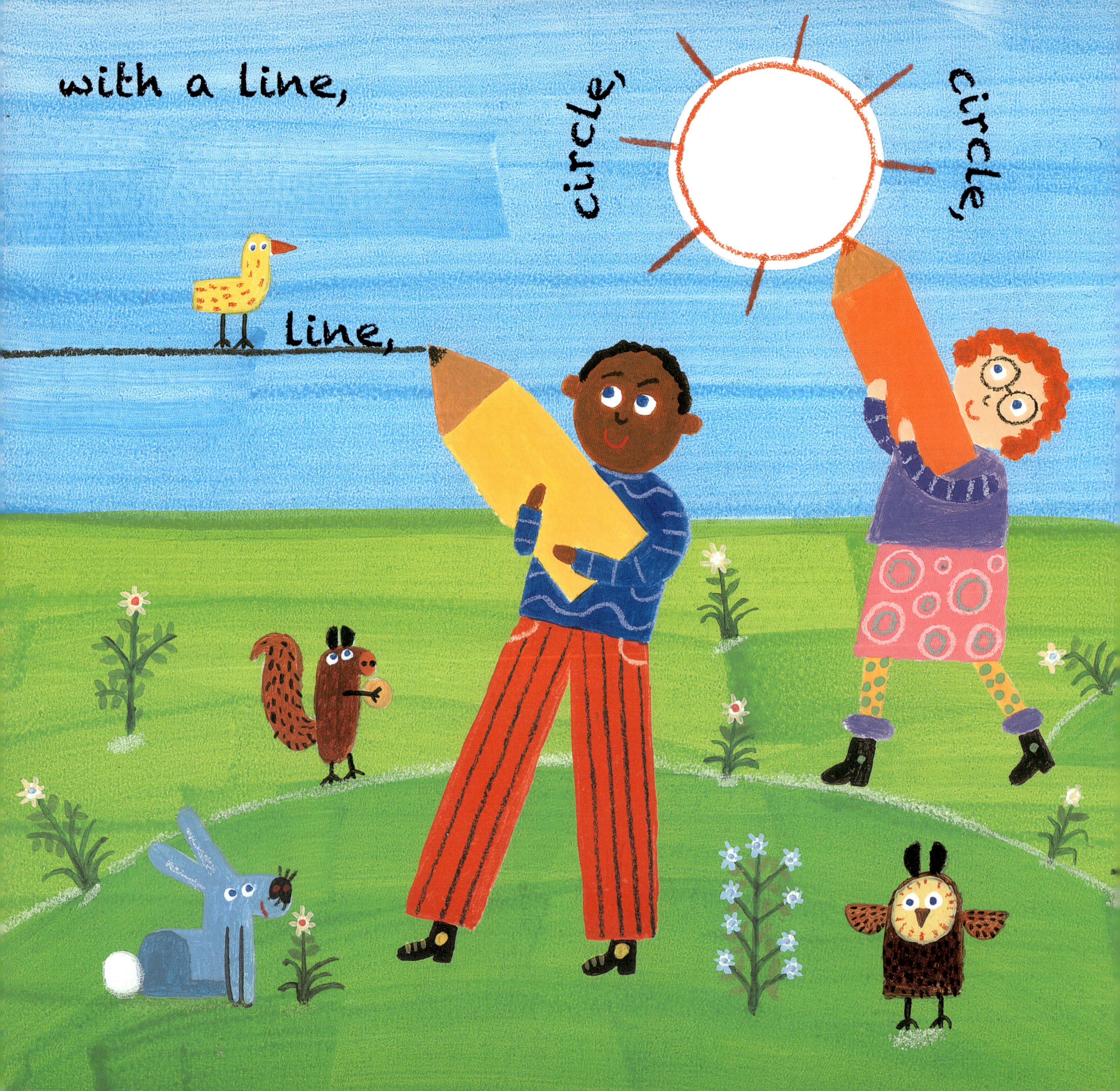

with a line,
line,
circle,
circle,

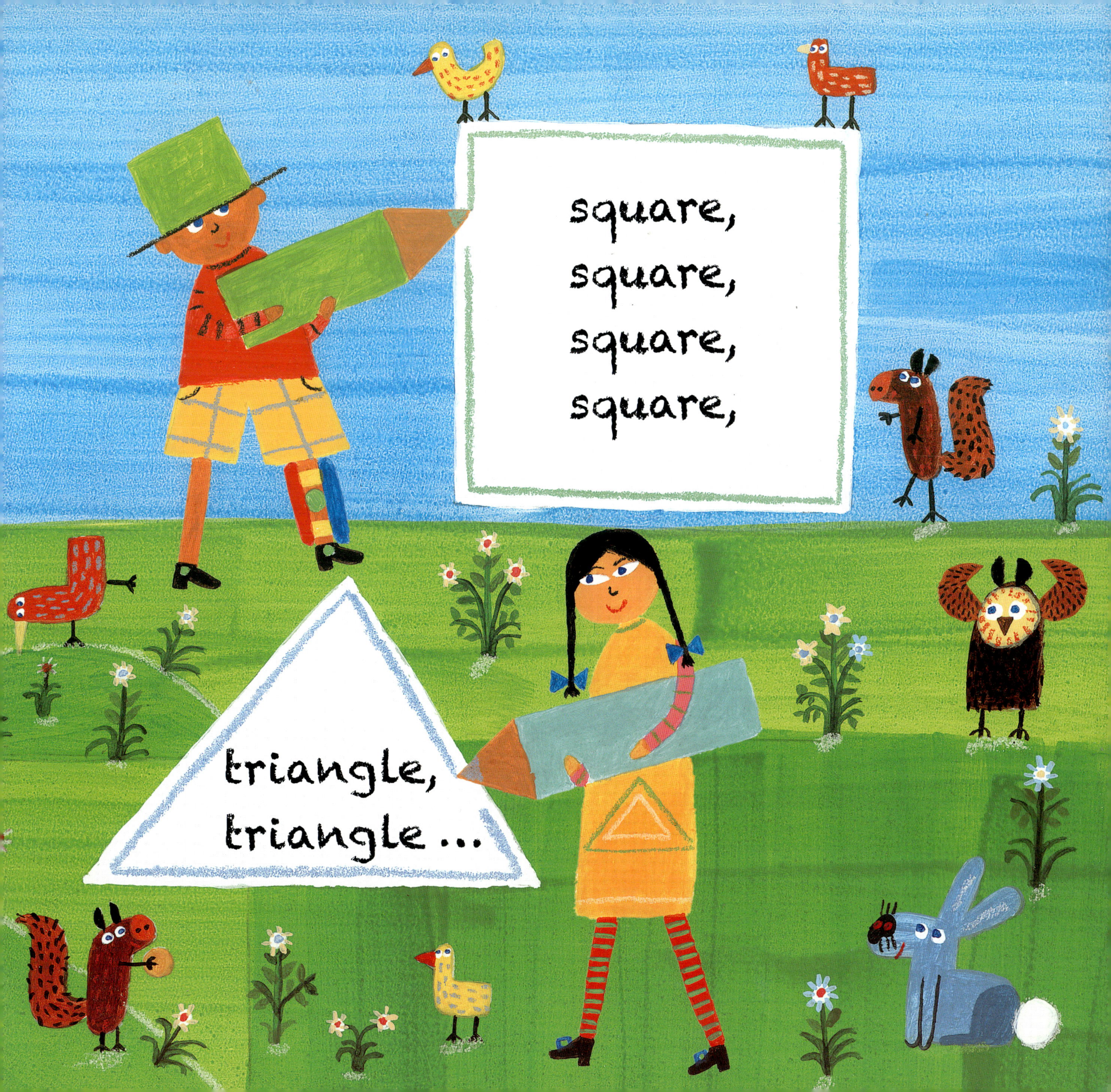
square,
square,
square,
square,
triangle,
triangle ...

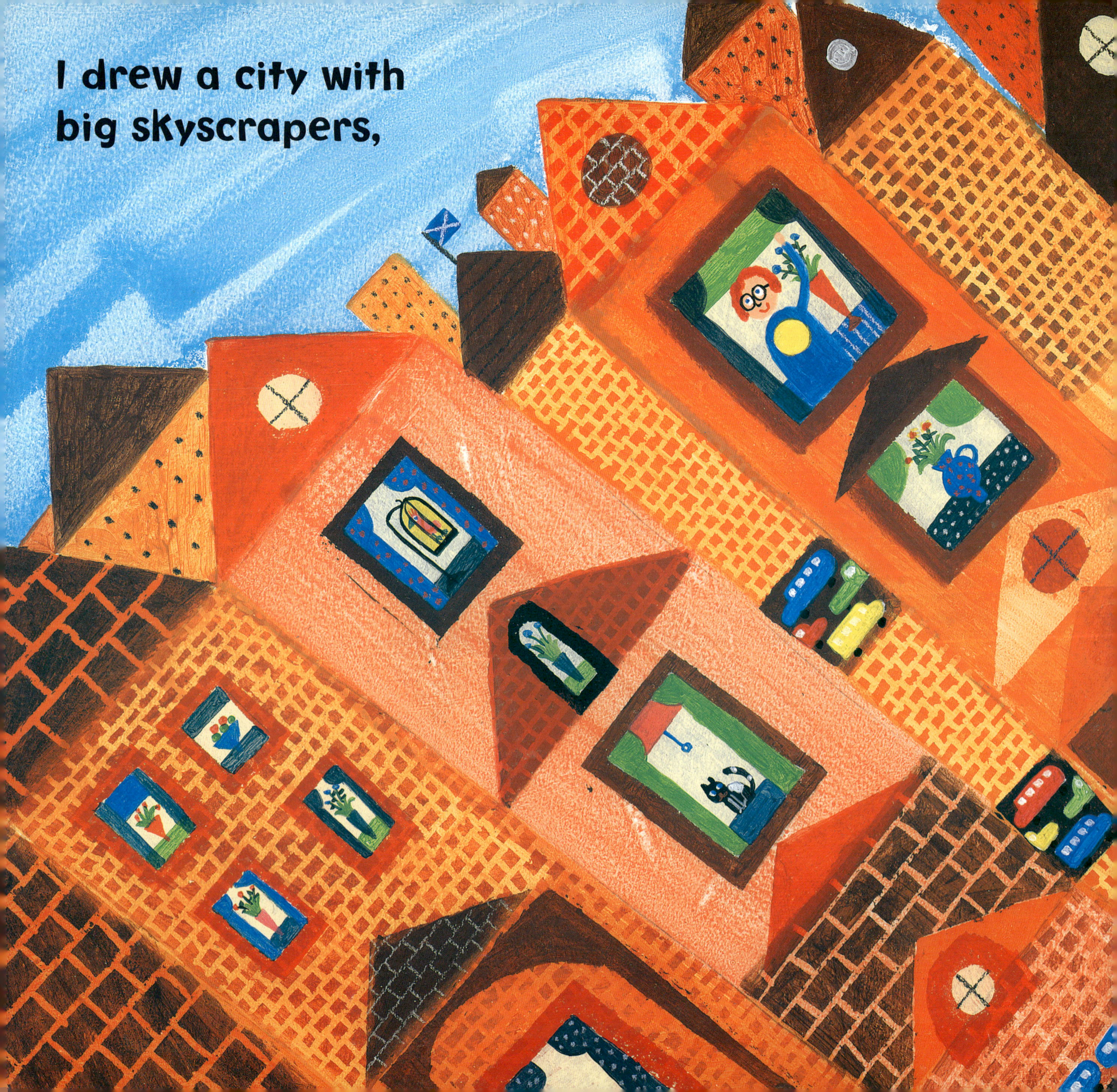
I drew a city with
big skyscrapers,

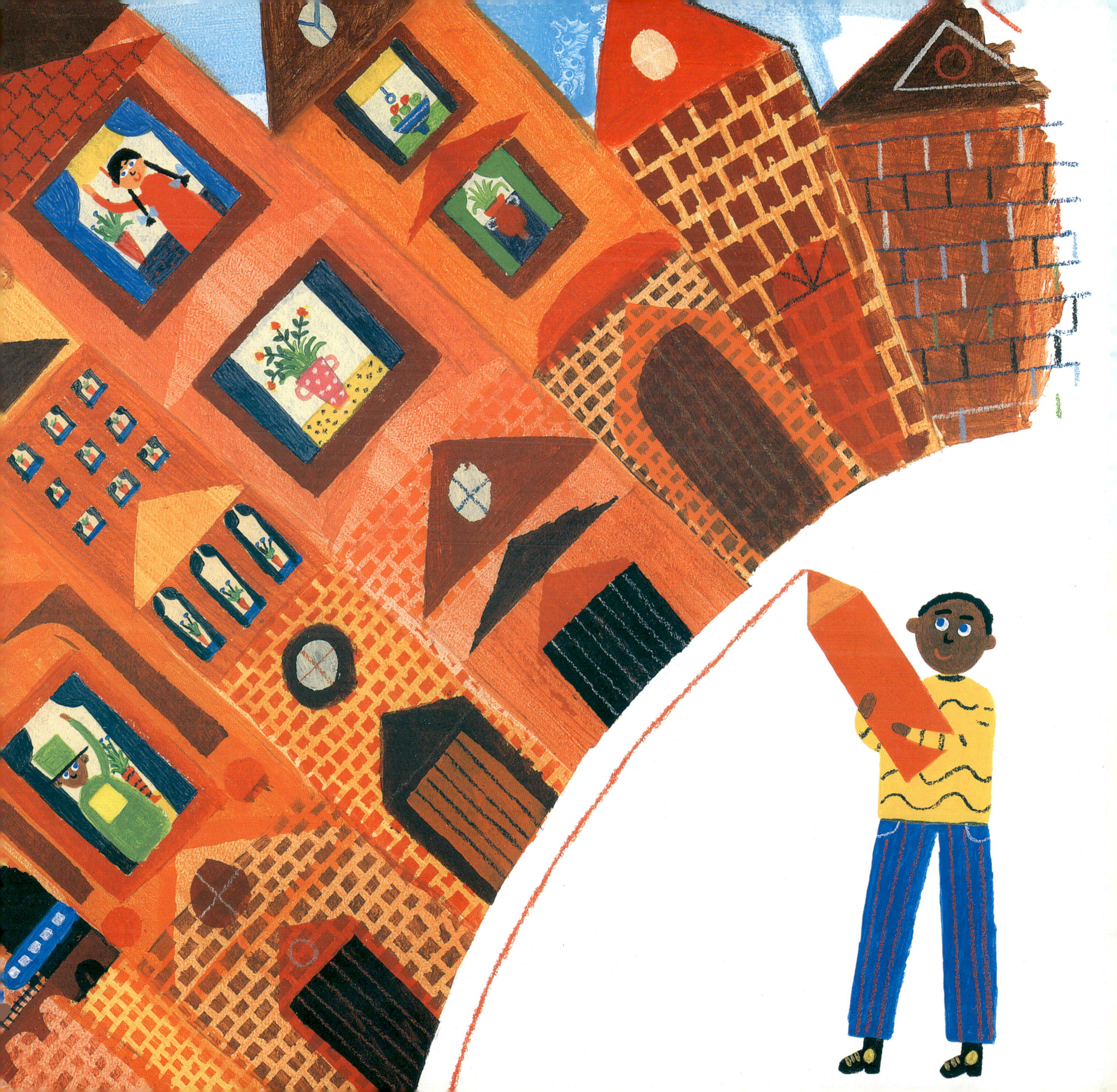

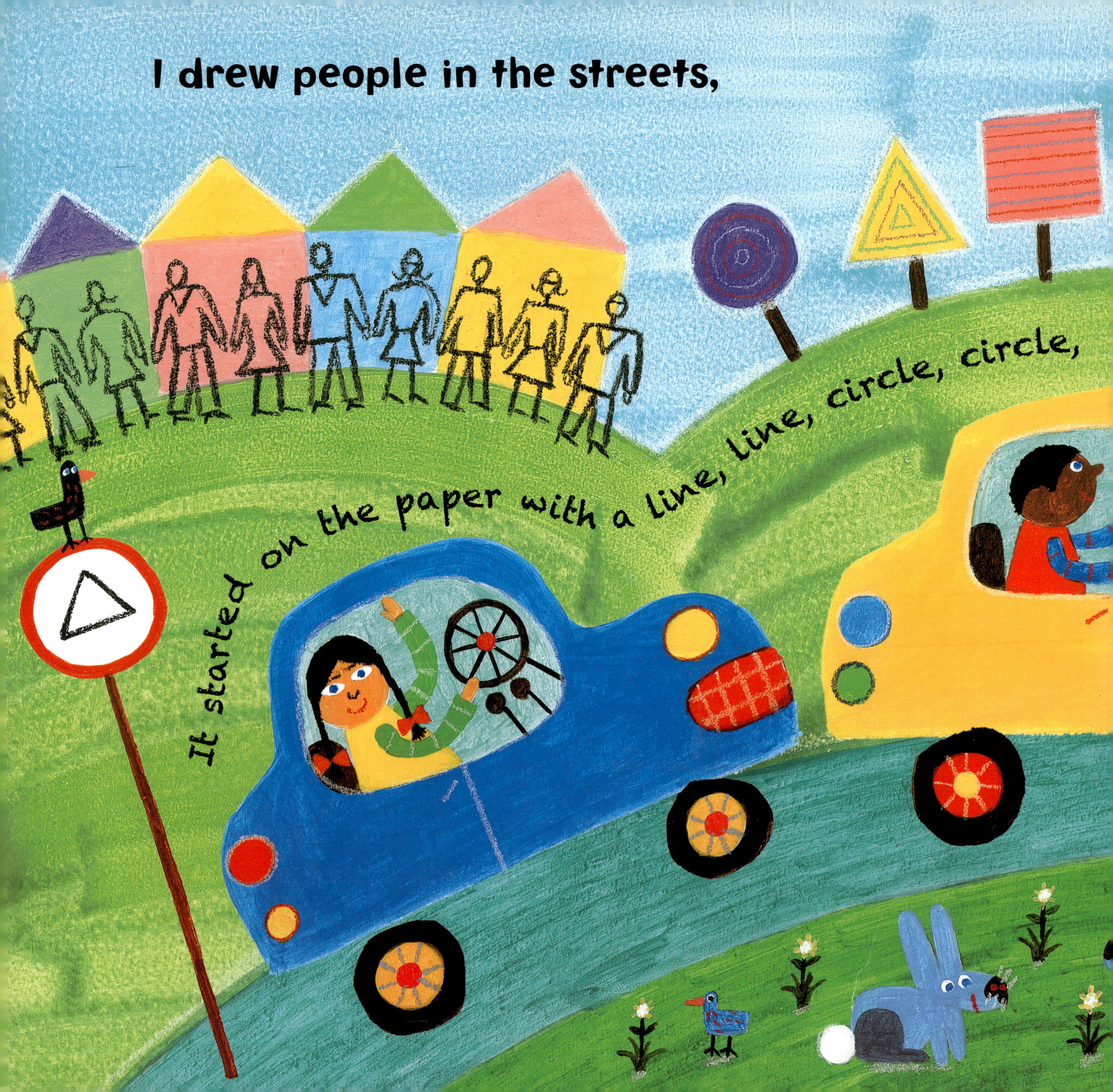
I drew people in the streets,
It started on the paper with a line, line, circle, circle,

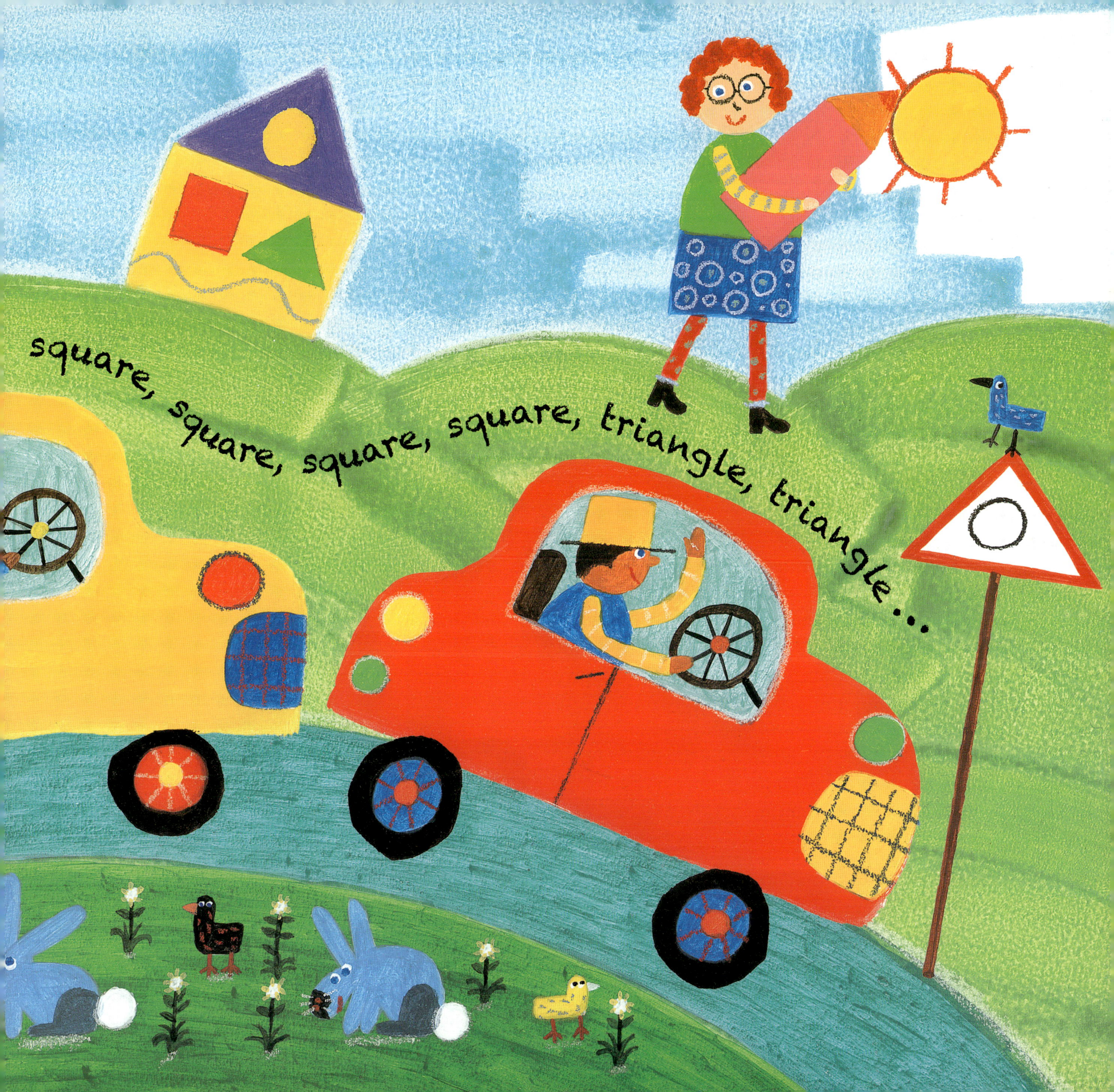
square, square, square, square, triangle, triangle...

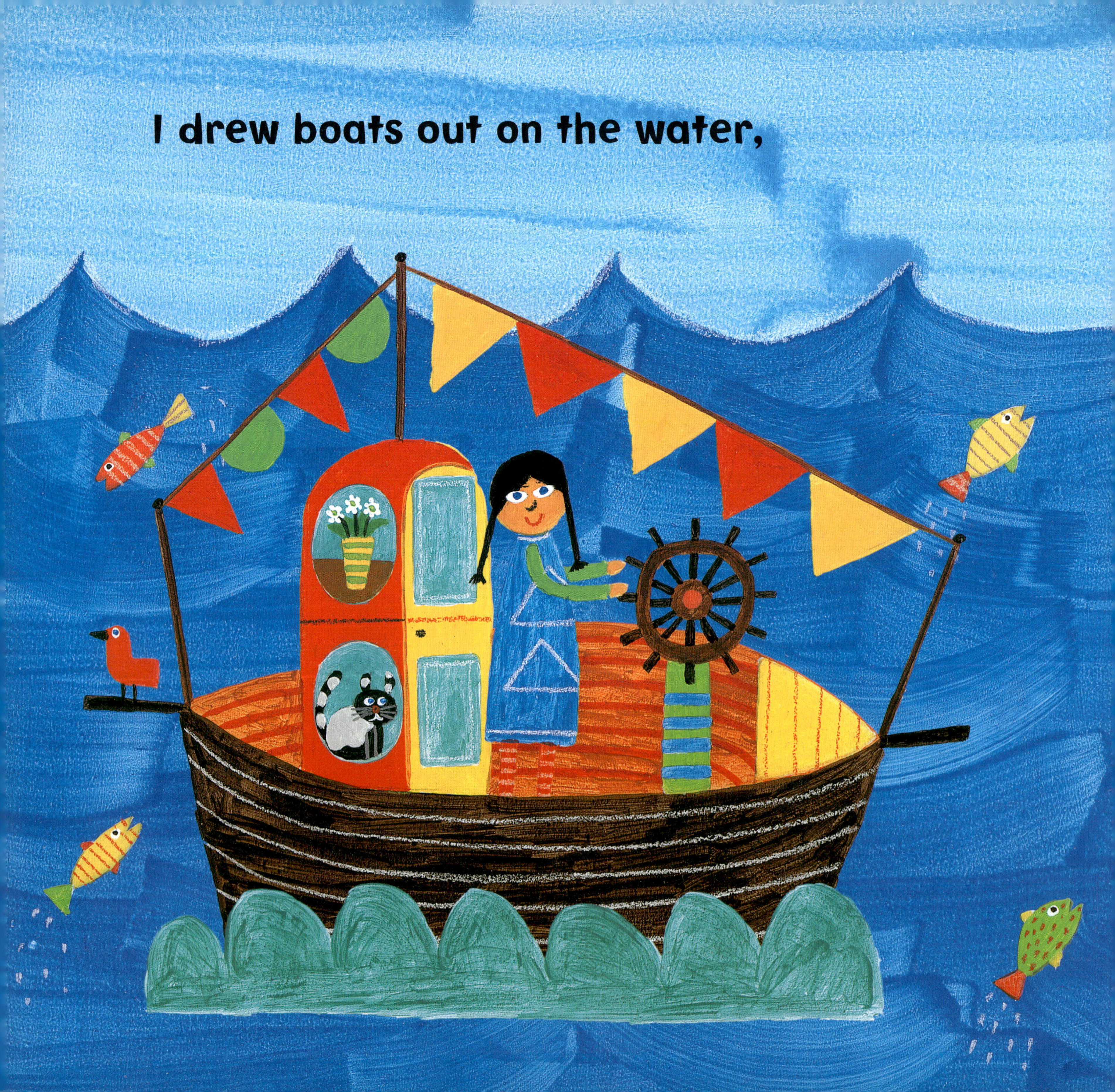
I drew boats out on the water,

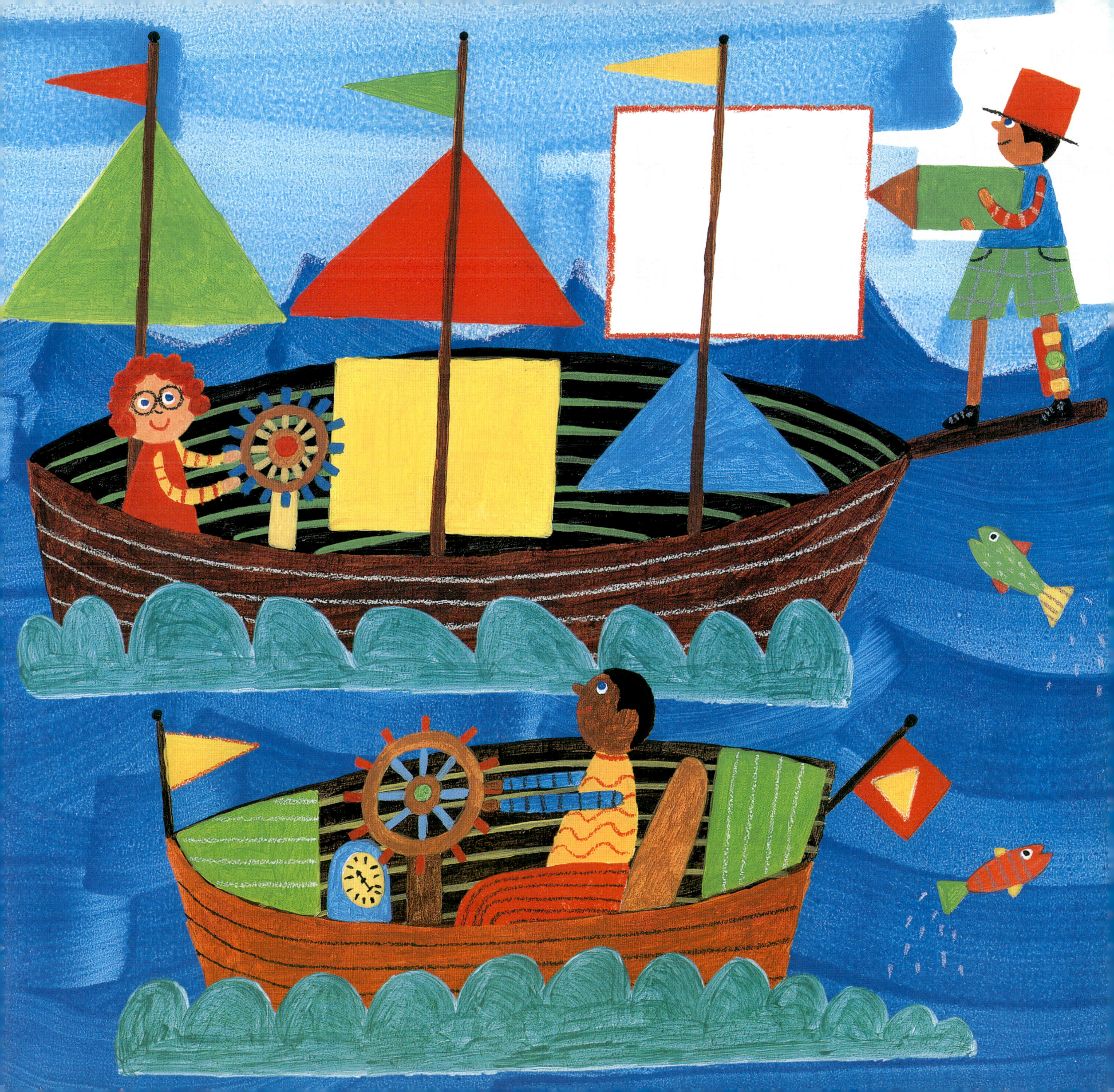

I drew a castle on the sand,
I drew a beachside waterslide,
Oh, what a ride!

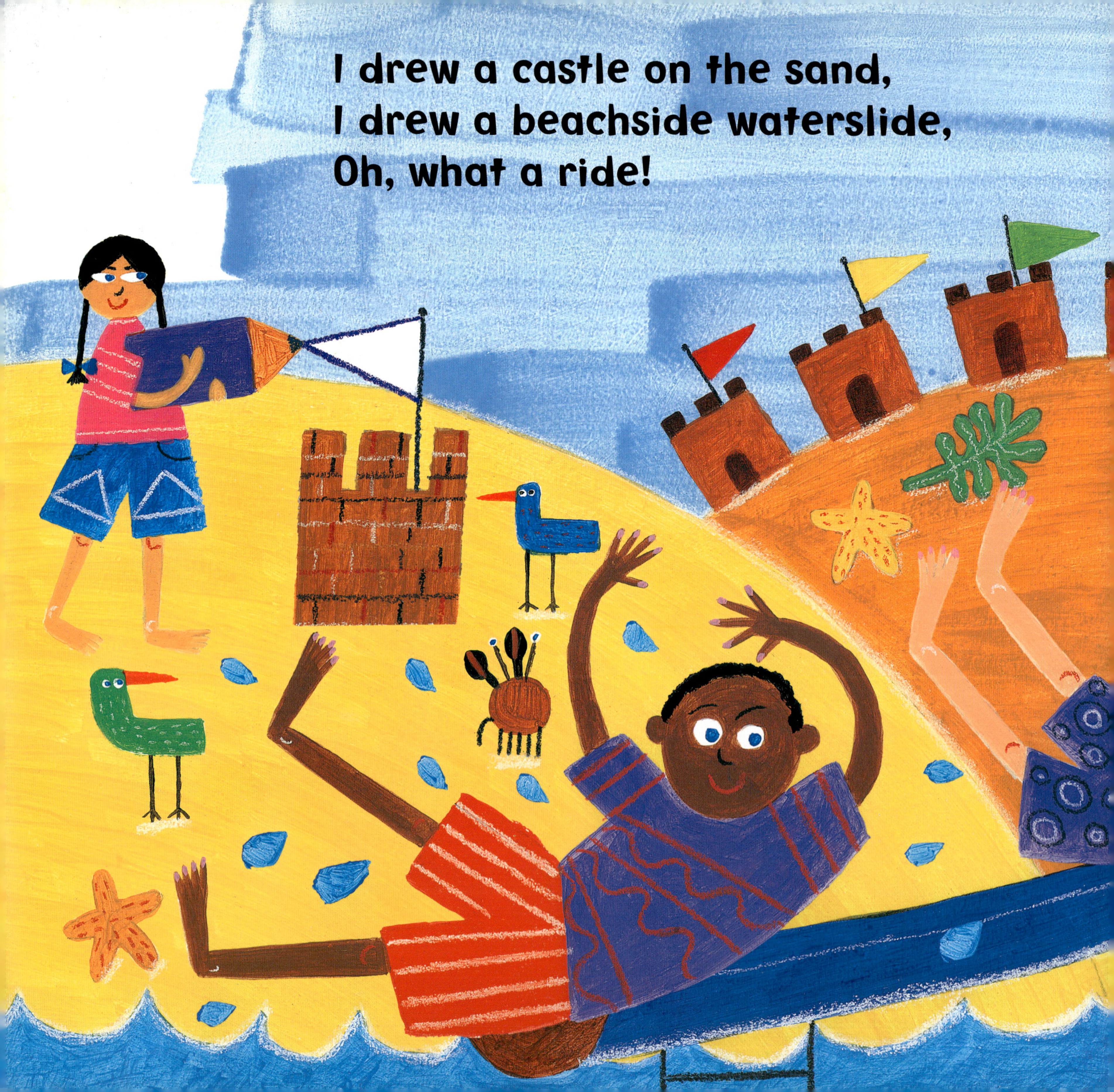

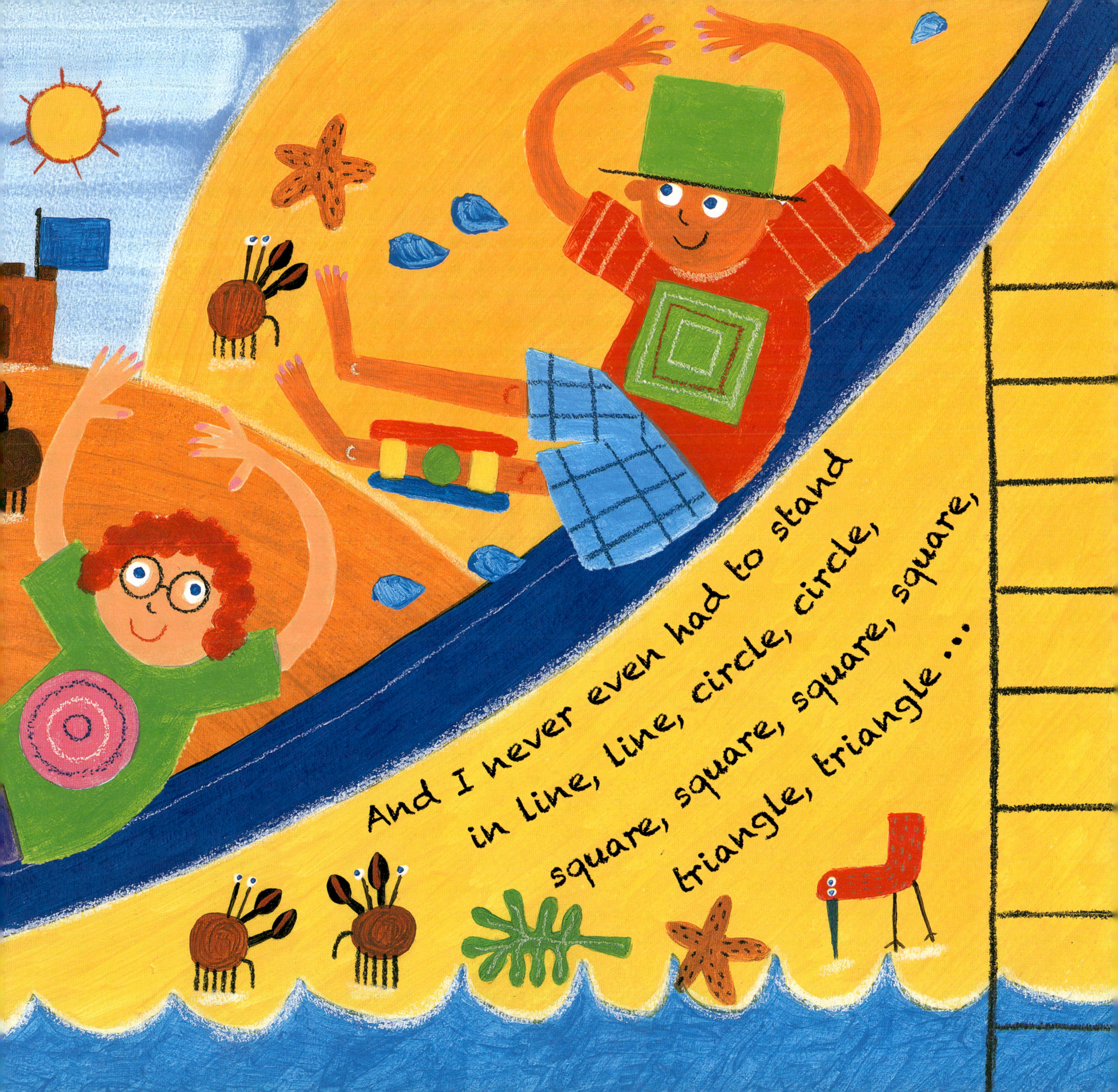
And I never even had to stand
in line, line, circle, circle,
square, square, square, square,
triangle, triangle ...

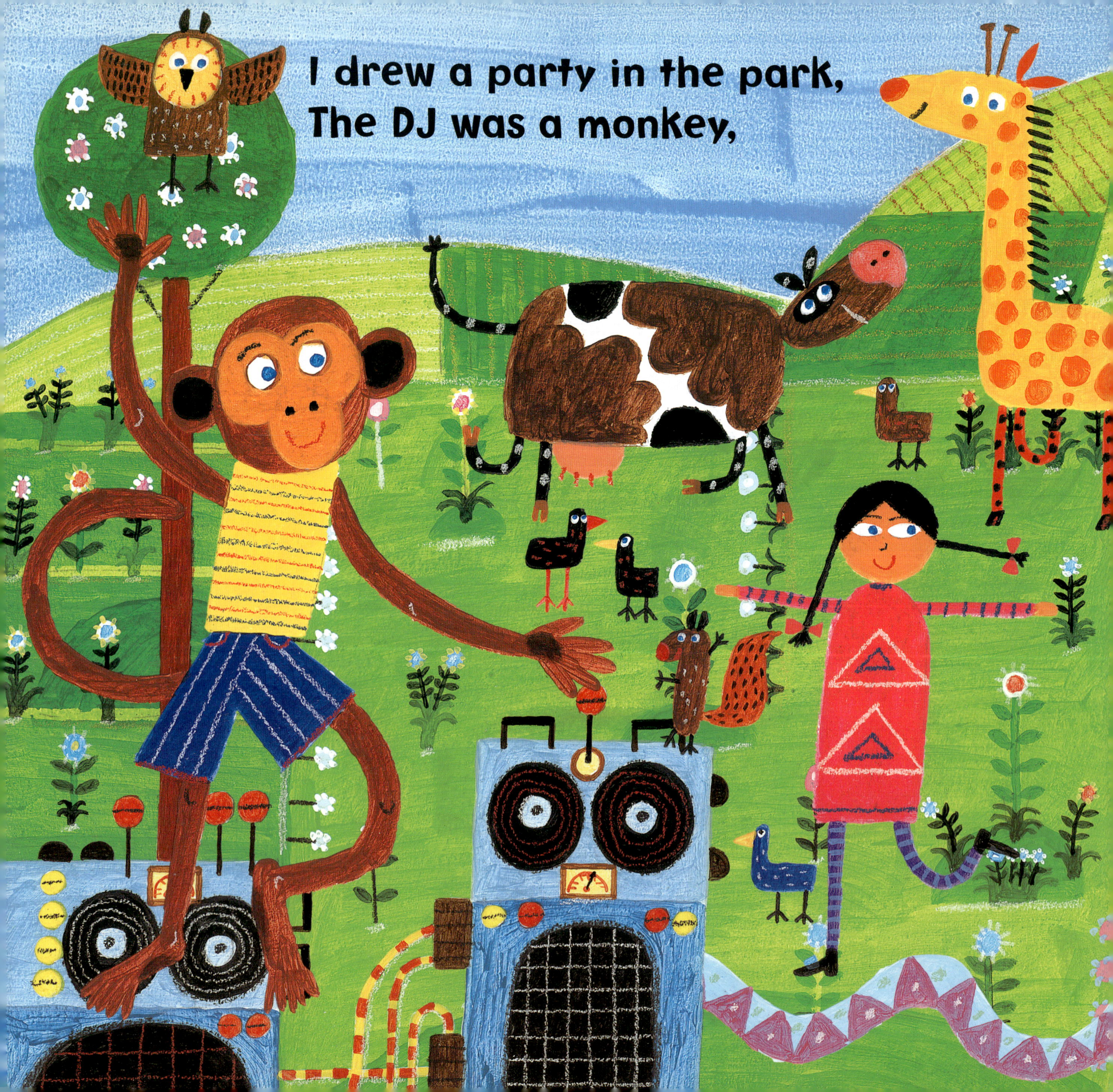
I drew a party in the park,
The DJ was a monkey,

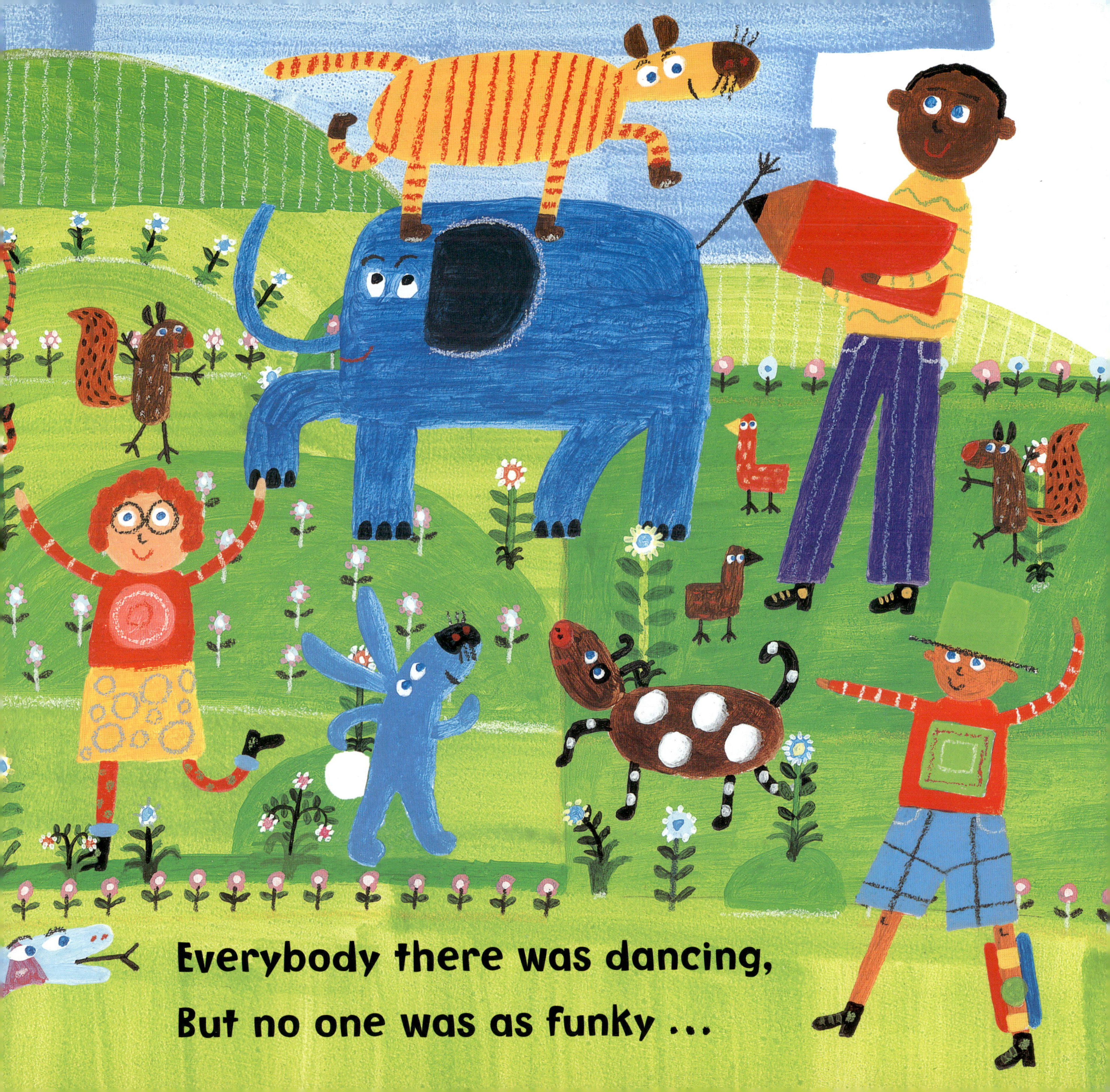

Everybody there was dancing,

But no one was as funky ...

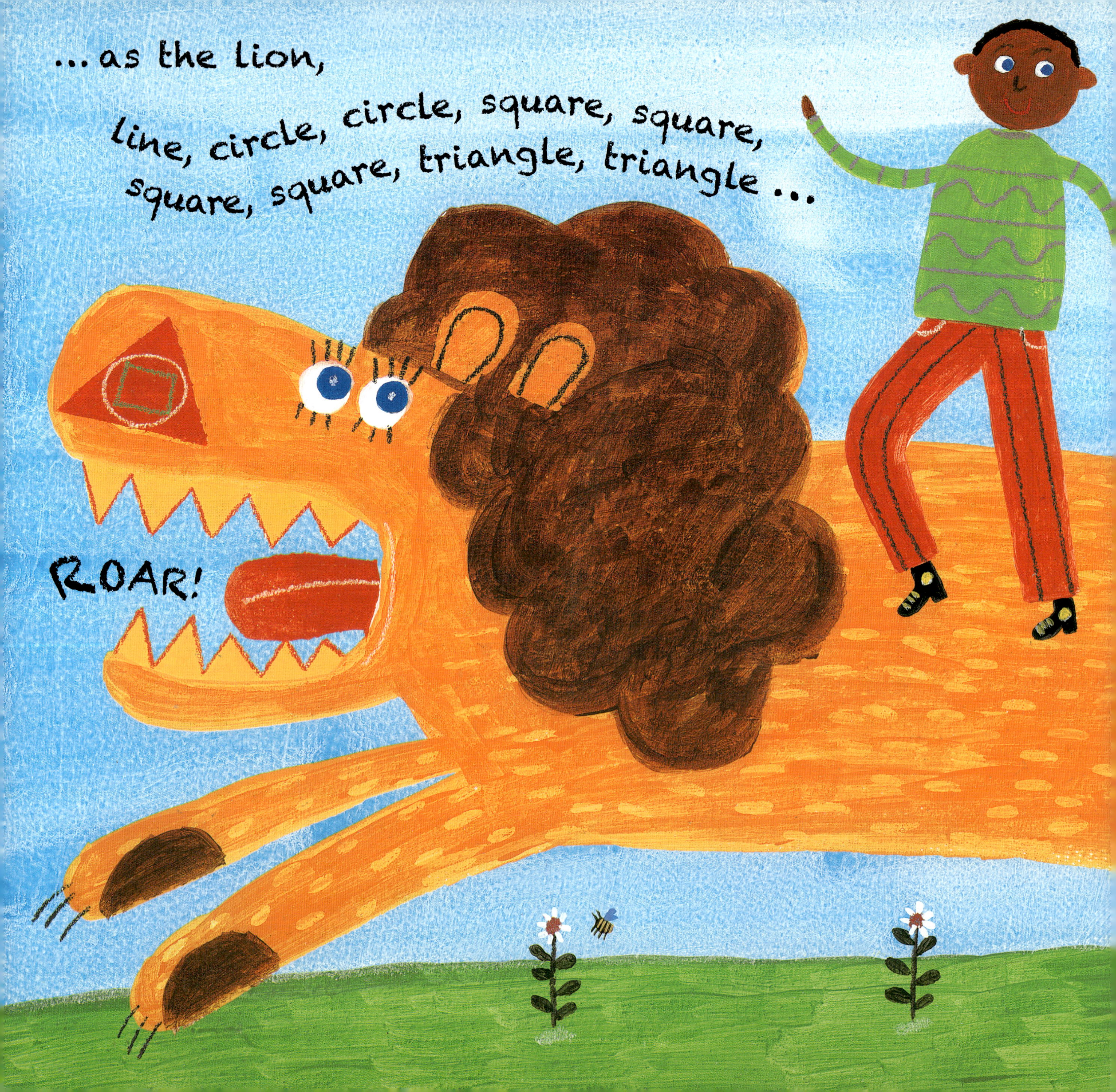
... as the lion,
line, circle, circle, square, square,
square, square, triangle, triangle ...
ROAR!

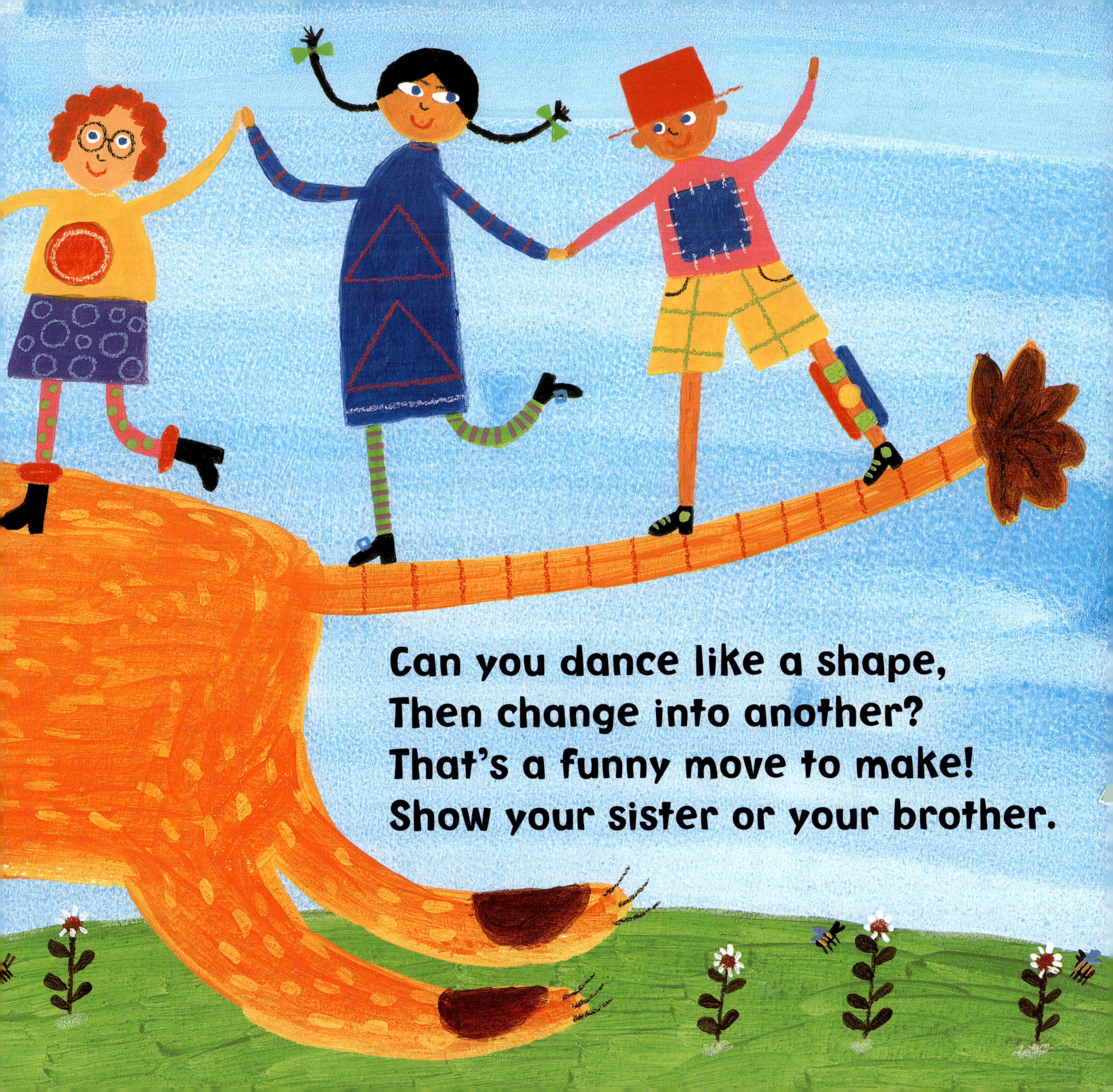

Can you dance like a shape,
Then change into another?
That's a funny move to make!
Show your sister or your brother.

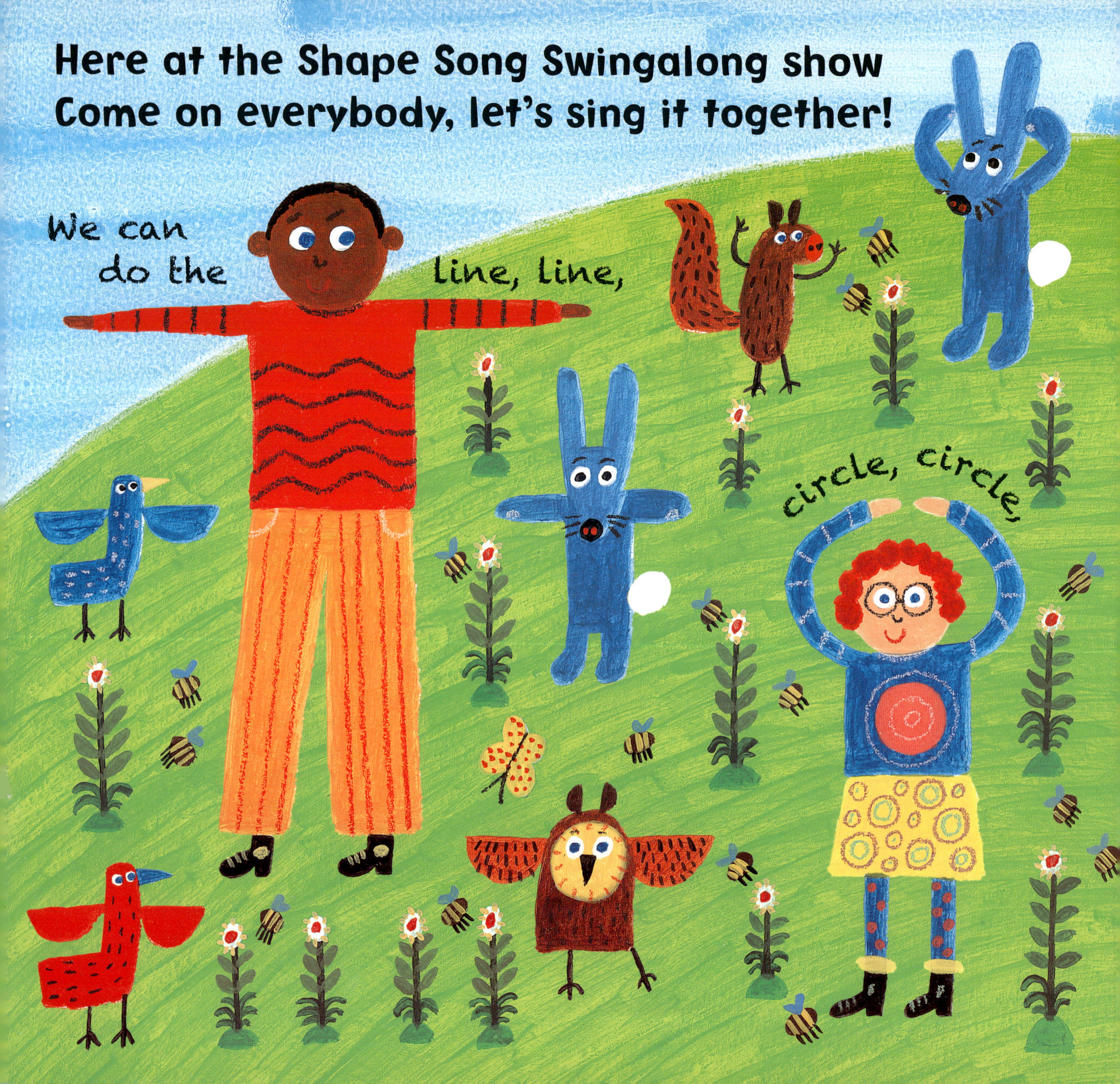
Here at the Shape Song Swingalong show
Come on everybody, let's sing it together!
We can do the
line, line,
circle, circle,

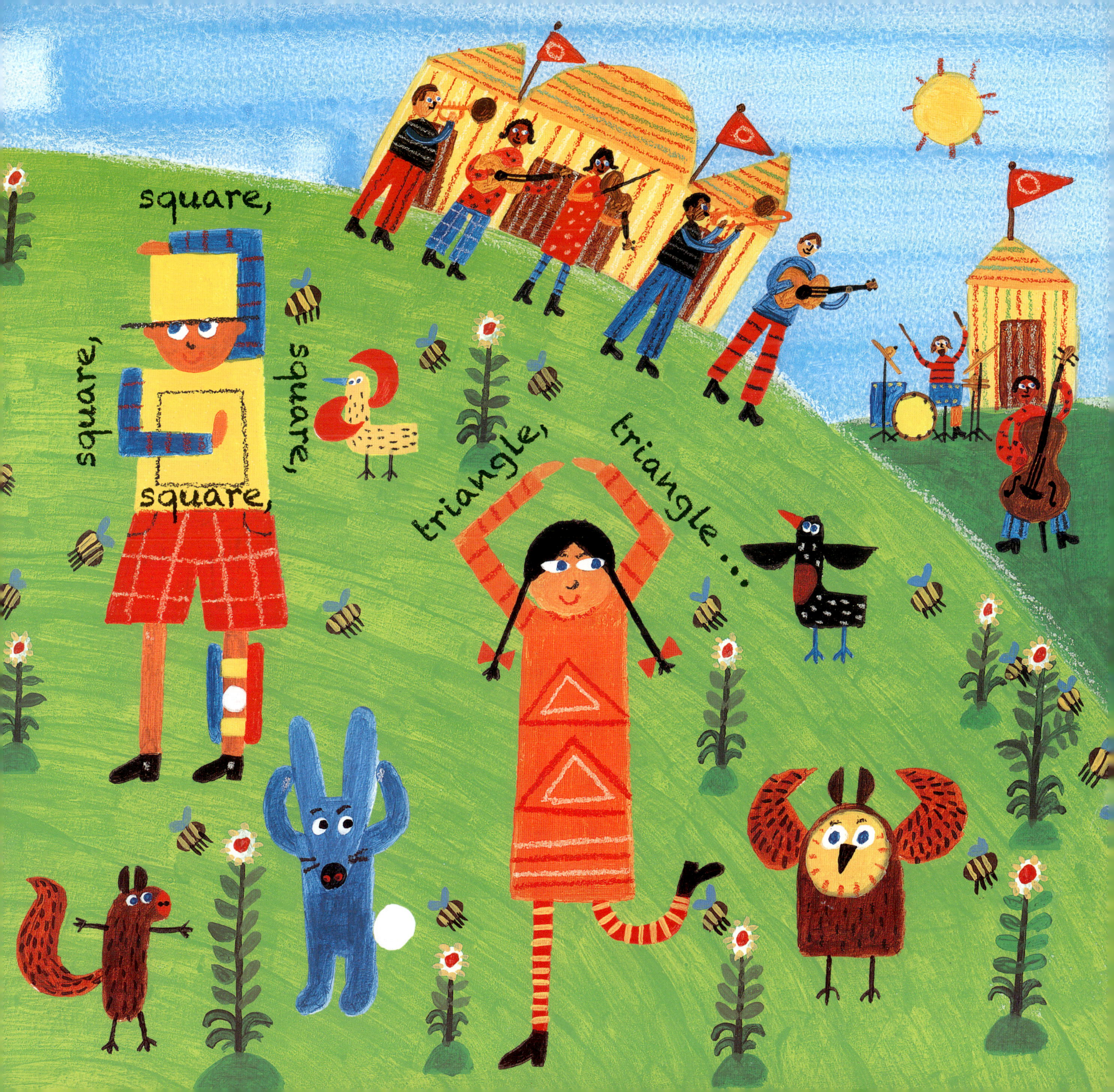
square,
square,
square,
square,
triangle,
triangle ...

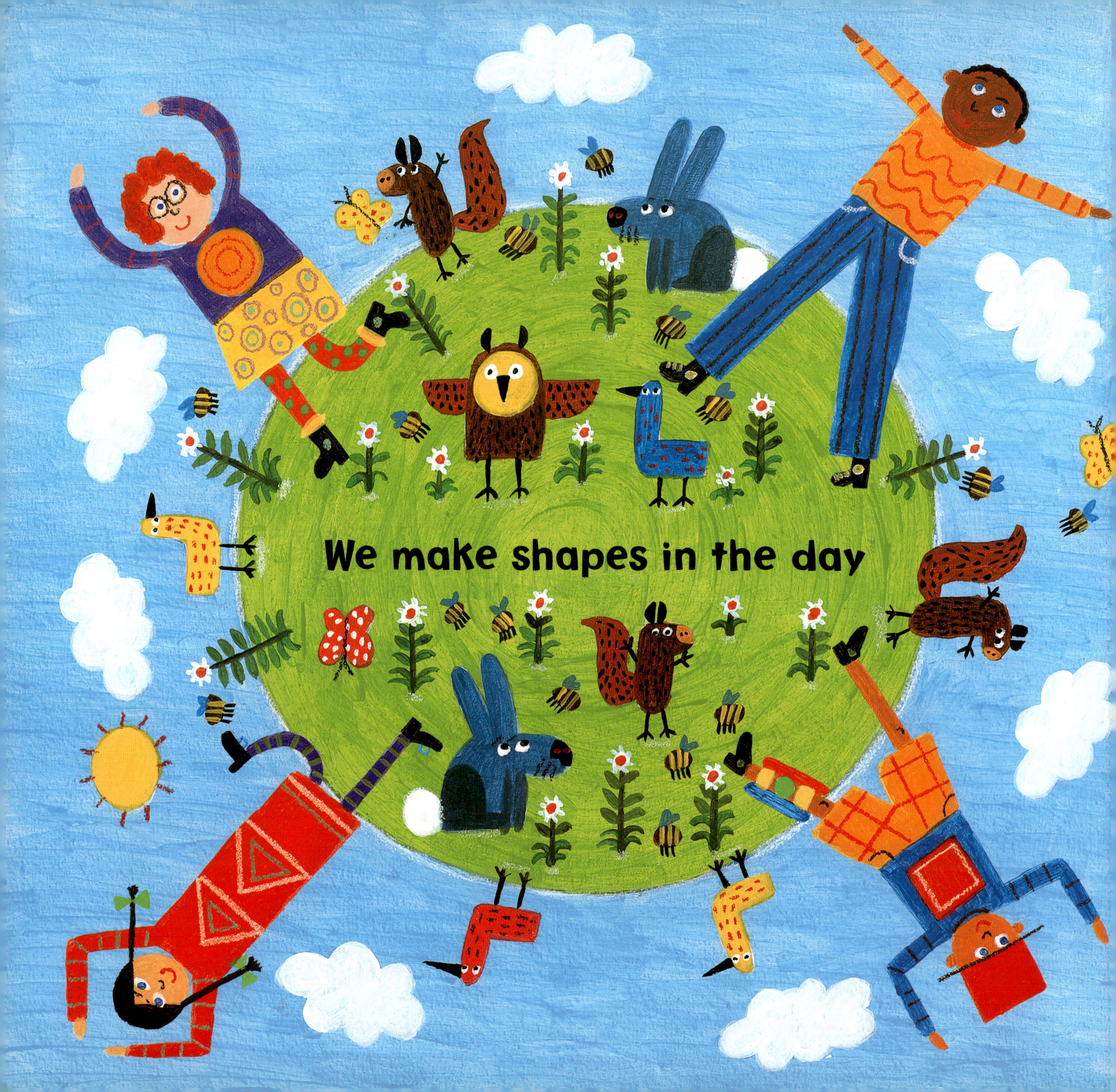
We make shapes in the day

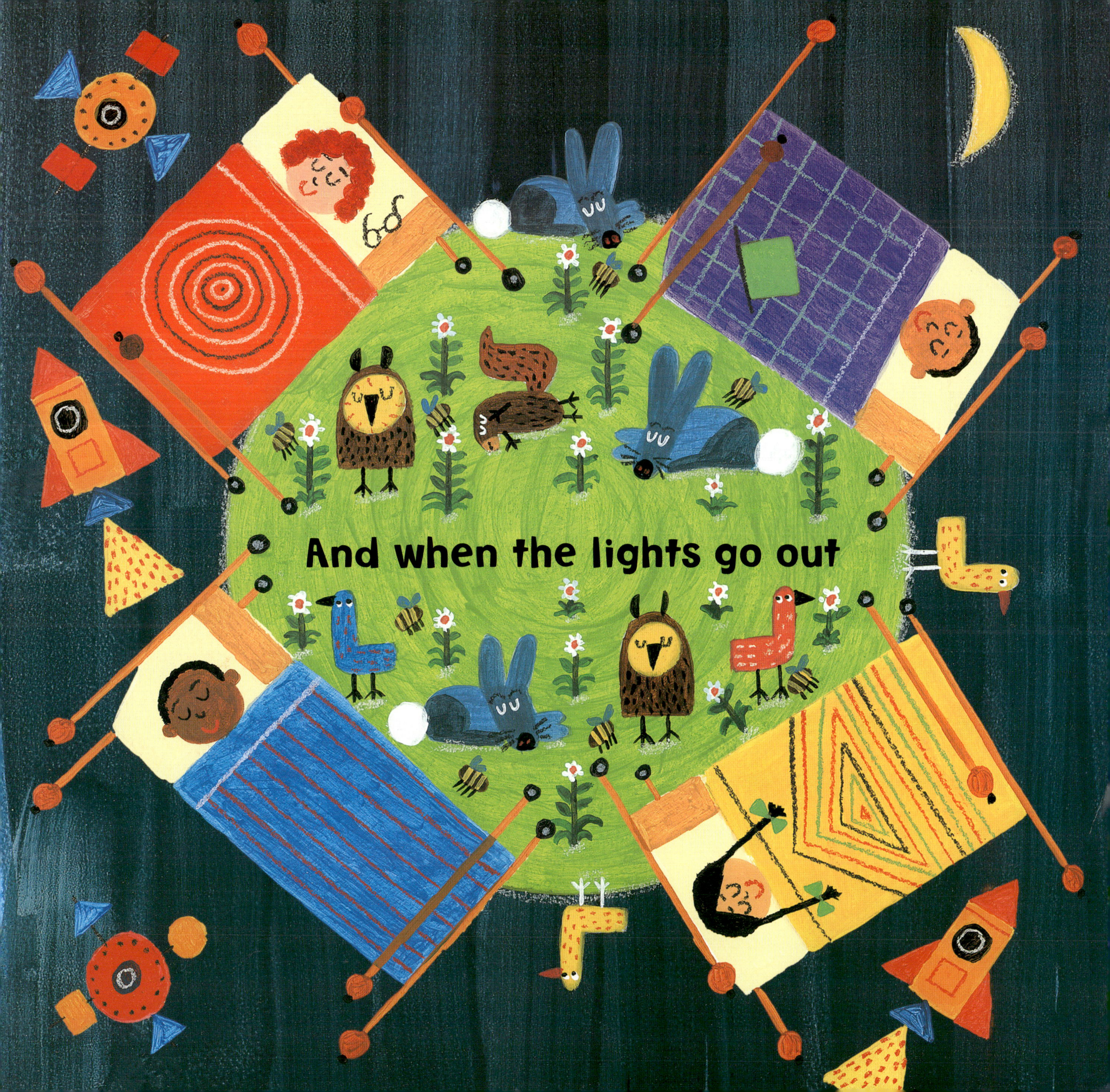
And when the lights go out

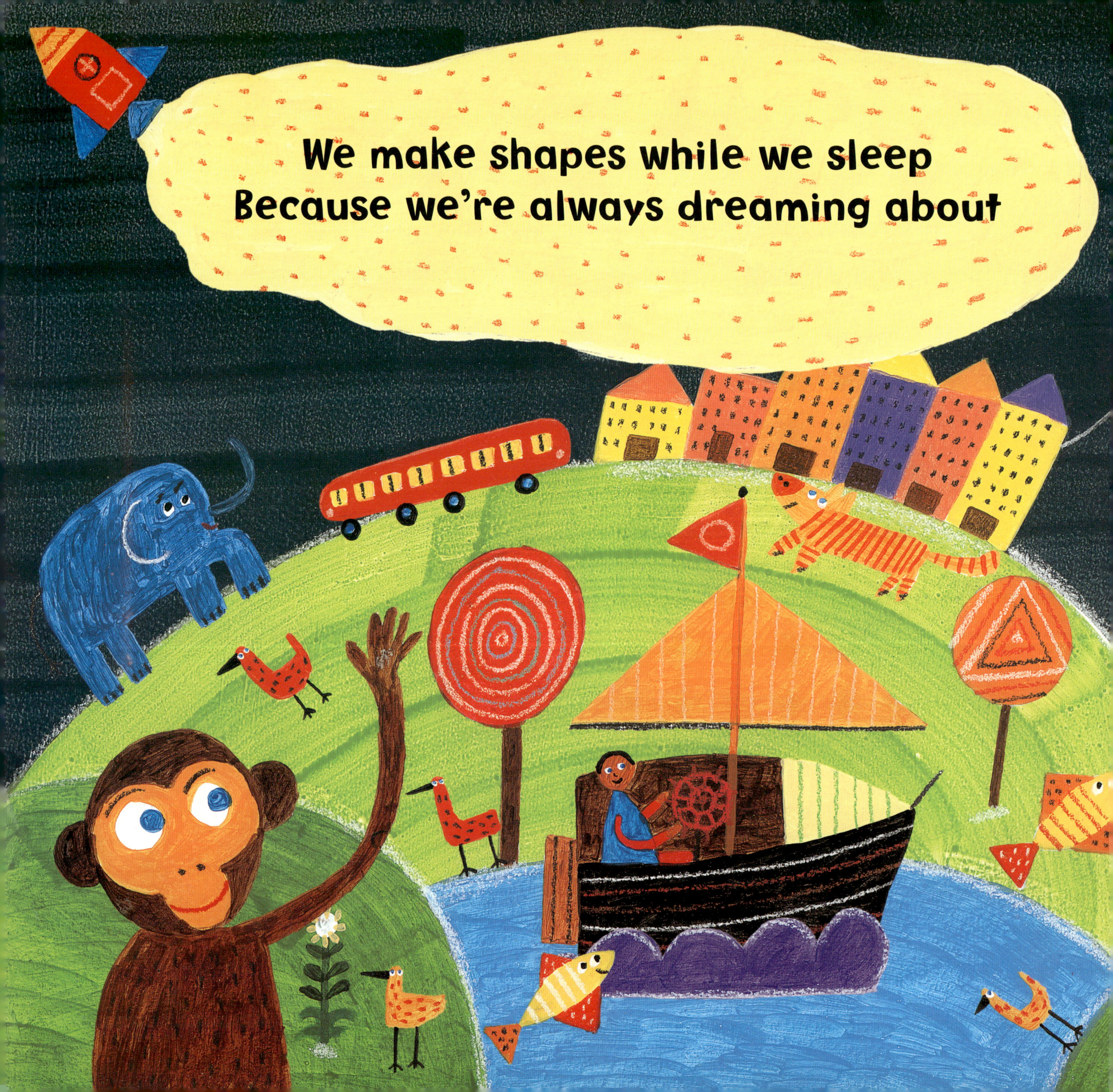
We make shapes while we sleep
Because we're always dreaming about

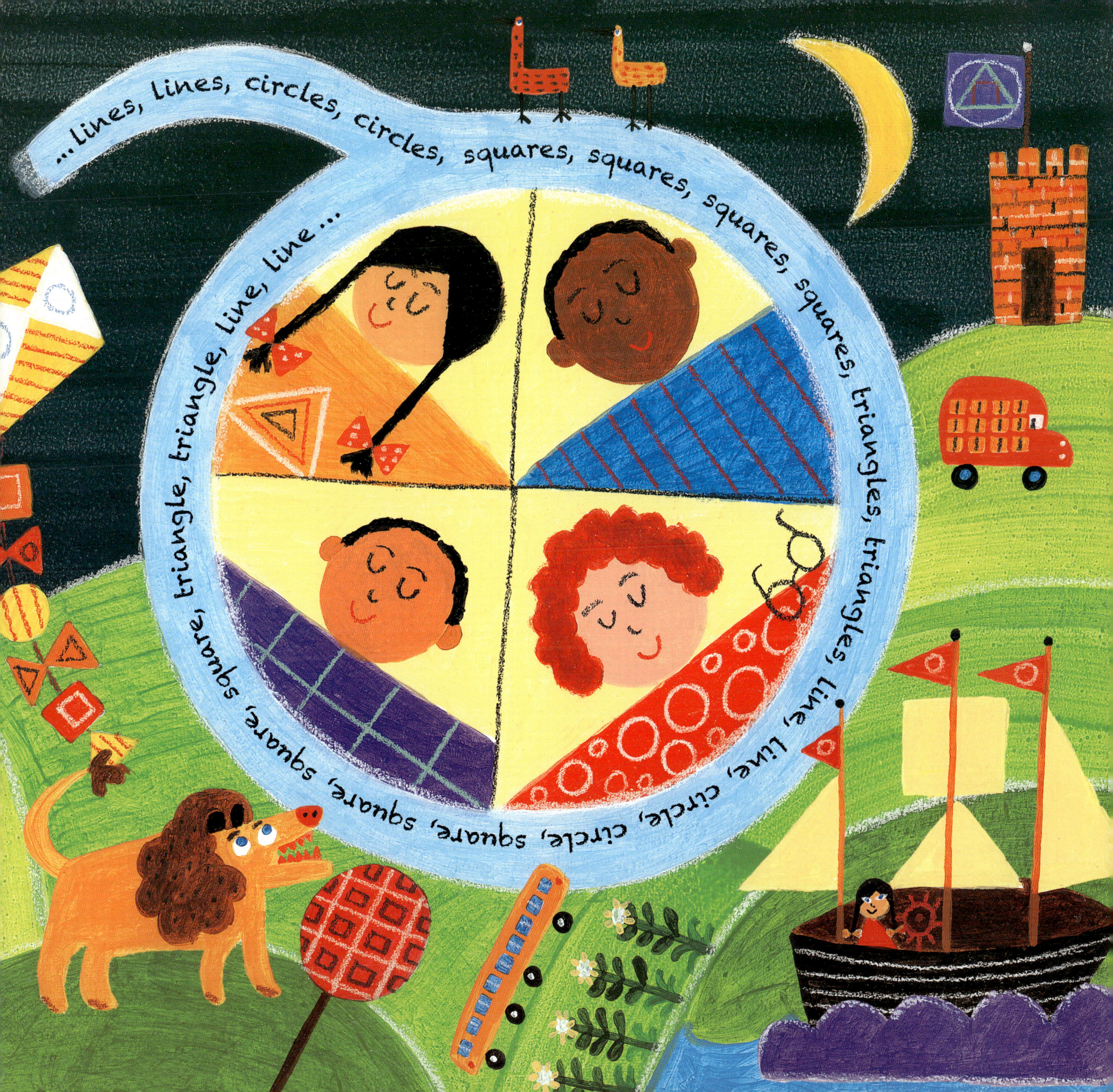
...lines, lines, circles, circles, squares, squares, squares, squares, squares, triangles, triangles, line, line, circle, circle, square, square, square, square, triangle, triangle, line, line, line...

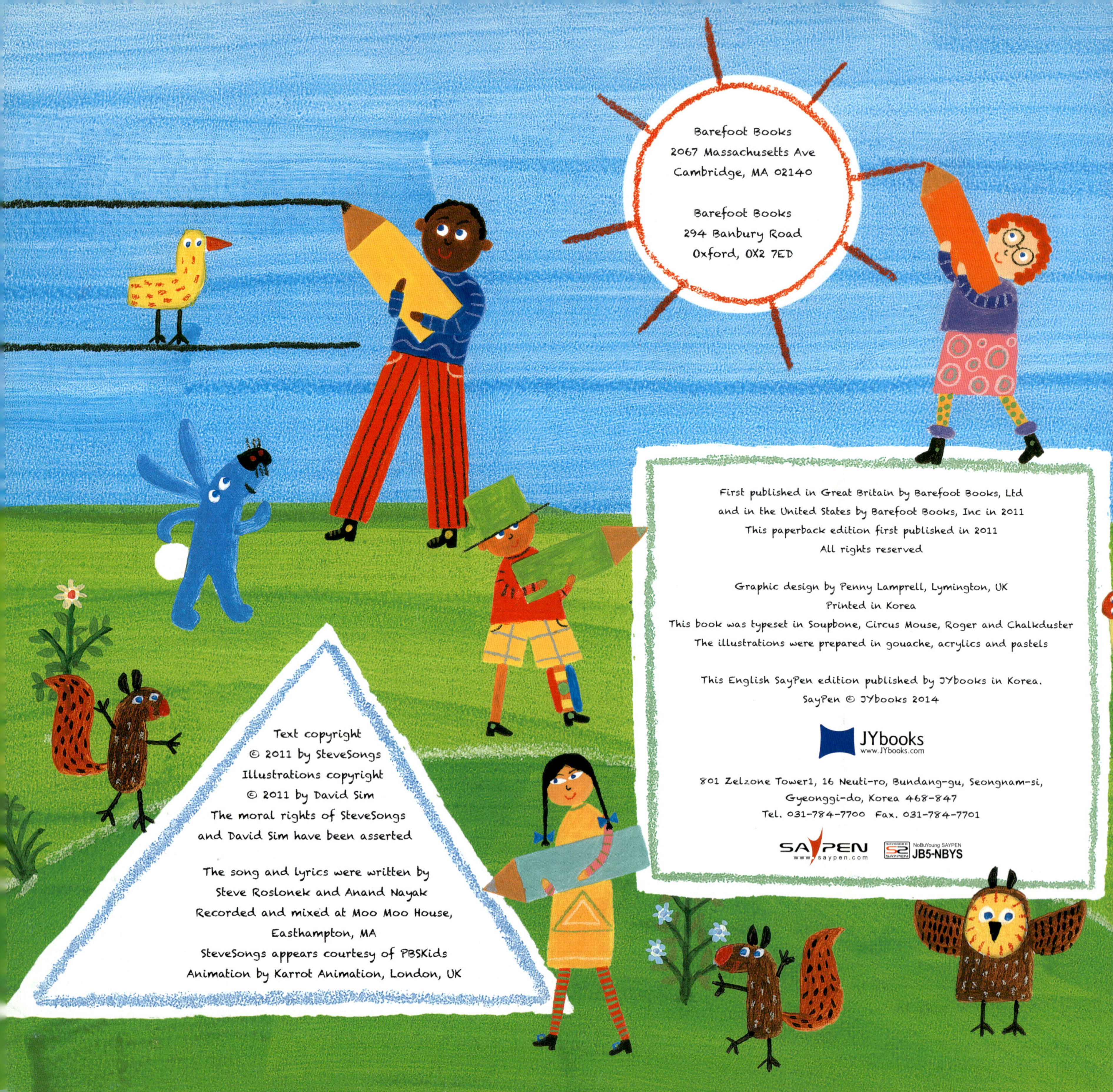
Barefoot Books
2067 Massachusetts Ave
Cambridge, MA 02140

Barefoot Books
294 Banbury Road
Oxford, OX2 7ED

First published in Great Britain by Barefoot Books, Ltd
and in the United States by Barefoot Books, Inc in 2011
This paperback edition first published in 2011

Graphic design by Penny Lamprell, Lymington, UK
Printed in Korea
This book was typeset in Soupbone, Circus Mouse, Roger and Chalkduster
The illustrations were prepared in gouache, acrylics and pastels

This English SayPen edition published by JYbooks in Korea.

JYbooks
www.JYbooks.com

801 Zelzone Tower1, 16 Neuti-ro, Bundang-gu, Seongnam-si,
Gyeonggi-do, Korea 468-847
Tel. 031-784-7700 Fax. 031-784-7701

SAYPEN
www.saypen.com
NoBuYoung SAYPEN
JB5-NBYS

The song and lyrics were written by
Steve Roslonek and Anand Nayak
Recorded and mixed at Moo Moo House,
Easthampton, MA
SteveSongs appears courtesy of PBSKids
Animation by Karrot Animation, London, UK